Clear Skin From Within

A 9 Step Guide on How to Eliminate Acne For Good

By Brigitte Bell

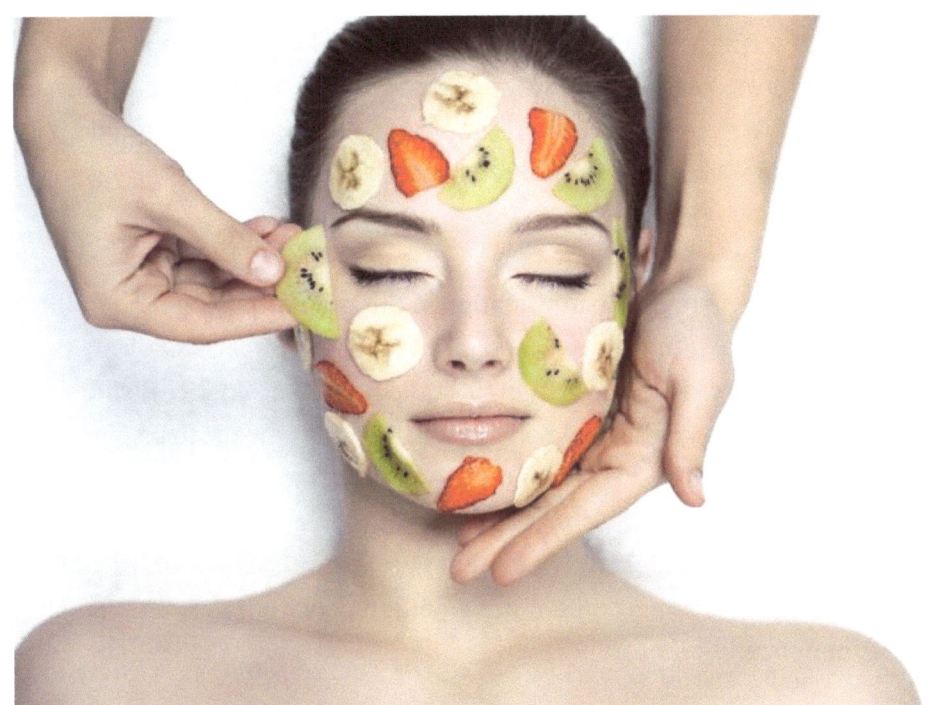

Clear Skin From Within

A 9 Step Guide on How to Eliminate Acne For Good

By Brigitte Bell

Copyright © April 30, 2015 — Brigitte Bell

Publication date: May 1, 2015

Cover image: Shutterstock.

Printed in the United States of America

Table of Contents

"If somebody has got beautiful skin, it invites us to a deeper understanding of what is going on inside their body."

-David Wolfe, Hungry For Change Film

Where there is health, there is beauty.

My Battle with Acne

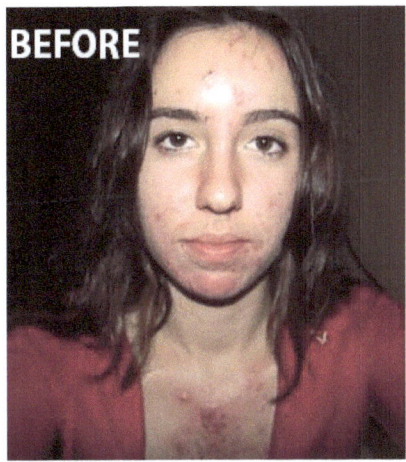
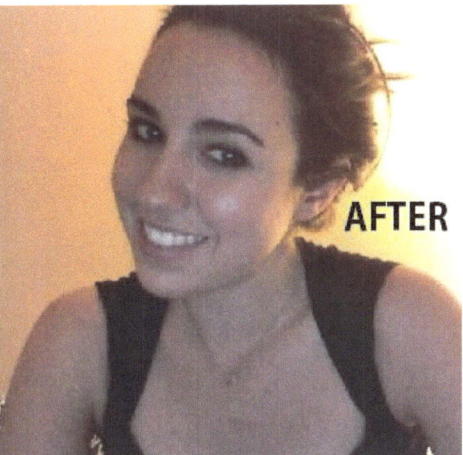

To those who knew me in High School, they also knew struggling with acne was one of my biggest battles. It seemed to me that no matter what I tried to do to have clear skin, no matter how many topical ointments I attempted to use, that nothing would rid me of my problem with poor skin. To those of you who have struggled with acne, like me, you know first-hand how emotionally and physically painful dealing with such an issue can be. My face and chest were covered in cysts that sometimes came in the size of quarters. But it wasn't until one day when I had two different teachers at my high school ask me if I was going to "do anything" about my poor skin condition that I hit rock bottom. Despite how painfully embarrassing this moment was for me, it was also the biggest blessing; because it was at that particular moment that I decided I would no longer struggle with acne, and that I was going to do anything and everything within my power to find the cure for clear skin. Which is what brings us here. I struggled for years, so that hopefully, you don't have to. My journey and research has led me to discover what causes acne and other skin conditions, and what we can do to naturally fix it. The body is an amazing machine, and given the right "fuel," and conditions, it will heal itself.

Components of Clear Skin

The first thing I'd like to establish in this book is that *Clear Skin Comes from Within*. Treating acne solely by external means is only treating the symptom of a much deeper, root problem. Acne is a symptom with a root cause of possible toxicity, hormone imbalance, stress, poor digestion, an imbalanced blood sugar, poor immunity, or even parasitic infestation. Therefore, treating acne solely by topical means would be like stuffing tissue paper in your nose to prevent your nose from running when you have a cold. Yes, your nose may stop dripping, but you've done nothing to treat the actual cold, which requires that you get rest and build up your immunity. So it is the same with treating acne. If we desire clear skin, we must begin from within.

I've comprised this book into 9 different sections, all of which are crucial in addressing if one desires to have clear skin. In Step 1 I'll share with you the importance of detoxing and supporting a healthy digestion and liver function. Step 2 will be about healing the gut, improving the body's elimination of waste, and ridding the body of unwanted visitors (parasites) that could be the cause of your poor skin, and how to re-inhabit the body with the "good" bacteria necessary for having healthy skin. In Step 3, I'll share with you the role hormones play in maintaining clear skin, and a few things you can do to help naturally balance them (This will be beneficial not only to your skin, but to those of you struggling with PMS as well). In Step 4 I'll discuss why it's important to Balance your Blood Sugar, and what you can do to accomplish that. In Step 5 I'll discuss the vital role having a healthy immune system, and what you can do to boost your immunity. In Step 6 I'll share with you some of my most powerful "Secret Weapons" when it comes to having clear skin. I'll discuss natural herbs, supplements, and remedies you can use to begin having flawless skin. In Step 7 we'll address the vitally important role Diet and Lifestyle factors play in having clear skin. I'll share with you the optimal diet for clear skin, and how other lifestyle factors such as exercise and having a healthy form of stress management will help you achieve and maintain the skin of your dreams! In Step 8 I'll discuss the importance of balancing your body's and skins pH levels, as to create the perfect environment for clear and healthy skin. Finally, in Step 9, I will share with you a few tips for external care of your skin. I share this information last, because as I mentioned before, contrary to what most believe is the secret to clear skin, clear skin comes from within, and is something that must be treated *internally* in order to gain lasting results. Are you as excited as I am to begin this journey?! I cannot wait for you to learn these invaluable gems of information so that your days of suffering may be O V E R!

Let's begin, shall we? ;-)

The Herxheimer Reaction

One more thing I'd like you to be wary of before we begin is the Herxheimer reaction. The Herxheimer reaction is a very common, normal occurrence that happens when the body is killing off toxins and eliminating harmful waste. When anyone makes the efforts to cleanse, heal, and detoxify their body, it's not uncommon for them to experience things like headache, sore throat, joint and muscle pain, sweating, chills, and cold or flu-like symptoms. Your skin may also initially feel a little more inflamed as well. In other words, you may feel a little worse before you begin feeling better. Don't let this alarm or discourage you from sticking with this protocol for clear skin. The fact that you may experience these symptoms on your journey is a positive sign that your efforts are working, and that you're well on your way to clear skin and having a toxin-free body. In fact, if you do experience any of these symptoms, you should feel glad that it's a testament to how much your body needed to detox in the first place. That being said, remember that if you begin experiencing any of these symptoms, it's a normal sign that fungus, bacteria, and parasites are dying off, and that you should stick with your efforts in achieving clear skin if you want to fully heal.

What is Your Skin Telling You?

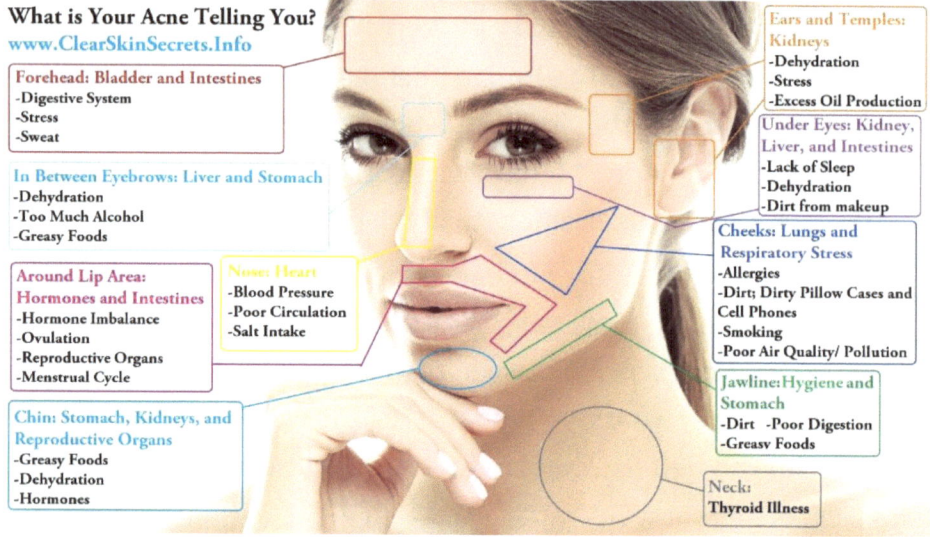

What is Your Acne Telling You?
www.ClearSkinSecrets.Info

Forehead: Bladder and Intestines
-Digestive System
-Stress
-Sweat

In Between Eyebrows: Liver and Stomach
-Dehydration
-Too Much Alcohol
-Greasy Foods

Around Lip Area:
Hormones and Intestines
-Hormone Imbalance
-Ovulation
-Reproductive Organs
-Menstrual Cycle

Nose: Heart
-Blood Pressure
-Poor Circulation
-Salt Intake

Chin: Stomach, Kidneys, and
Reproductive Organs
-Greasy Foods
-Dehydration
-Hormones

Ears and Temples:
Kidneys
-Dehydration
-Stress
-Excess Oil Production

Under Eyes: Kidney,
Liver, and Intestines
-Lack of Sleep
-Dehydration
-Dirt from makeup

Cheeks: Lungs and
Respiratory Stress
-Allergies
-Dirt; Dirty Pillow Cases and
Cell Phones
-Smoking
-Poor Air Quality/ Pollution

Jawline: Hygiene and
Stomach
-Dirt -Poor Digestion
-Greasy Foods

Neck:
Thyroid Illness

Ancient Chinese medicine teaches that when it comes to acne, each area of our break-outs are indicative of a certain bodily system failing. This is incredibly useful knowledge to have as it helps us pinpoint the true source of our acne and individualize treatment by targeting the specific cause. Rather than just trying a bunch of different remedies and hoping that one works, we can accurately self-diagnose by simply looking at our face in the mirror and identifying the precise origin and root source of our blemishes. Once we know the true cause of our acne, we can then take action towards fixing the bodily system that is causing it. Take a look at the chart above and see if you identify with any of the problems associated with the acne you're experiencing in a particular region of your face.

Upper Forehead: Bladder and Intestines- If you have acne here, it is indicative of poor digestion, the build-up of toxins, as well as sweat.

Solution: Begin incorporating more antioxidants in your diet. Try green tea, berries, as well as the supplements I mention later on like Glutathione and Alpha-Lipoic acid.

Lower Forehead- Acne in this region shows there is an imbalance in the mind and spirit. You're likely suffering from stress, depression, or poor sleep habits.

Solution: Have a healthy form of stress management (which I'll get into more later), exercise to reduce stress, and be sure to get enough sleep.

Nose- Acne on the nose is a result of heart problems, poor blood pressure, and stress.

Solution: Exercise, rest, and get enough sleep. Have a diet that supports a health heart (avoids unhealthy saturated fats, etc.)

In Between Eyebrows- Acne in this region is likely a cause of excessive alcohol consumption, and a diet that is high in fat.

Solution: Avoid skin toxins, like alcohol. Cut out fats, and eat a diet that is full of fiber (to eliminate toxins) and nutrients.

Around the Lips- Acne around the lips is typically due to hormonal causes such as imbalances or being on a menstrual cycle. It could also be a sign of problems with the intestines, and/or constipation.

Solution: Have a test to get your hormones checked, or follow the protocol I reveal in the later sections as to what you can do for balancing hormones naturally. Be sure to have a diet that is fiber rich, full of fruits and vegetables, and drink plenty of water to help improve elimination.

Chin- Acne on the chin is usually a result of eating greasy or fast foods, dehydration, and hormonal imbalance.
Solution: Avoid greasy foods, drink plenty of water, and eat to balance your hormones (I'll teach you how in the later sections)

Ears and Temples- Acne on the ears and temples can be indicative of kidney problems likely due to a lack of water or too much salt and caffeine.
Solution: Drink plenty of water. Cut back on sugars, salt, and caffeine, as well as oil-producing foods.

Under Eyes — Acne under the eyes shows kidney, liver, and/or intestinal issues. It can also be a sign of lack of sleep, dehydration, toxicity, dirt build-up from makeup, or rubbing the eyes.
Solution: Get sleep, take care of your kidneys by drinking water and avoiding excessive caffeine, salt, sugar, alcohol, or any drugs. Take care of your liver through periodic detoxing and supplementing with herbs such as Dandelion and Burdock root, as well as Glutathione, Alpha- Lipoic Acid, and N-Acetyl Cysteine. Try to avoid putting on makeup or touching this delicate area.

Cheeks- Acne on the cheeks can be a result of allergies, smoking, pollution, or other respiratory stress.
Solution: Promote healthy lung function by avoiding smoking, getting out in fresh air periodically, and engaging in exercise to aide with proper respiratory function.

Jawline- Jawline acne is likely a result of poor hygiene and stomach issues.
Solution: Avoid foods that are incredibly processed as these are harder to break down for the stomach. Supplement with probiotics and digestive enzymes to aide with digestion. Change your pillowcase every other night, or sleep with a towel on your pillow to avoid the spread of bacteria. Avoid touching or picking at your face. Clean your cell phone regularly, try to avoid letting it touch your face—using the speaker phone or investing in a Bluetooth device or headphones can greatly help in the prevention of bacterial spread and growth.

Neck- Indicates a possible thyroid problem.
Solution: Eating a nutrient rich diet, full of fruits, vegetables, and leafy greens works to balance the thyroid.

As you may have probably already noticed, many of the causes for acne on various regions of the face overlap one another. For example, you may have notice that dehydration results in acne on the chin, eyebrows, ears, and temples. This is actually quite good news for you, because if you have acne on multiple areas of your face, you may begin to notice multiple areas of healing just by addressing one issue alone.

For example, improving digestion will help target the acne on the forehead, jawline, and under the eyes (a good digestion will help with ALL areas, but these ones specifically). Everything is interconnected and interrelated in the body. Once you begin to address one issue or bodily system, other systems begin to heal and balance out as well.

Step 1: Detox

One of the functions of the integumentary system (the skin) is to help the body eliminate waste. The skin, therefore, is an eliminative organ, meaning it will attempt to eliminate toxin, cellular byproduct, and other harmful waste via the epidermis (the top layer of the skin) thus resulting in issues like acne, psoriasis, and other skin disorders if there is a toxic build-up. The way to help get rid of acne is to first rid the body of toxins. One of the most powerful things I've ever done for my body was choosing to do a 5 day fast & cleanse. I purchased a cleanse kit from a local health food store. The kit included detoxifying herbal pills and a lot of fiber. When it comes to detoxing, it's important to stick with the cleansing for at least 5-7 days. The first 3 days are the most crucial, as it is during this time that most of the cleansing is taking place. The last 2-4 days after that are like maintenance, but still equally important as the first days. You don't want to start off your cleanse, decide it is too difficult, and then binge on Twinkies and nachos. It's important to carefully ease your body out of the cleansing stage to prevent your body from going into shock. To do an effective detox, you can purchase a cleansing kit at your local health food stores, or you can simply choose to do a fruit and vegetable cleanse, juice cleanse, or water cleanse. I'll go through each of these types of cleanses with you so that you can decide for yourself what you feel would be best for you. For those new to fasting and cleansing, it's probably best to start with the easier cleanses and work your way up towards the more difficult ones. Also remember to consult with your trusted health care professional before embarking on any major cleanse.

Fruit & Vegetable Cleanse

 A fruit and vegetable cleanse requires that one would only eat whole, raw fruits and vegetables for 5-7 days. This is ideal for someone who has never cleansed, and a good way to ease oneself into future deeper cleansing. During this time one can eat all the fruits and uncooked vegetables one desires. For breakfast, and ideal meal would be a fruit salad and fruit juice, and for the evening some salad and steamed vegetables.

Juice Cleanse

Doing a Juice cleanse requires that one drink only freshly juiced fruit and vegetable juices. While anybody can do this kind of cleanse, this type of cleanse is ideal for someone who already eats a healthy diet, and lives a relatively healthy lifestyle so that the detoxification process (the Herxheimer reaction) will be a little less intense and more bearable as compared to how it would be for someone who has a highly toxic lifestyle and body.

Water Cleanse

Water cleanses require that one only drink water for 5-7 days. This is a much more serious type of cleanse and it is definitely advised that you talk with your doctor before choosing to do such a cleanse.

Ending Your Detox

As I briefly mentioned before, the last days of your detox are as important as the first. You don't want to complete a detox only to gorge on a pizza and Pringles. End the first few days of your detox with a vegetable broth made from carrots and celery. Eat some carrots for your blood sugar, and celery for its water and fiber content. Drink freshly-made vegetable juices, and ease your way back into eating with salads, steamed vegetables, and potato.

Daily Cleansing

Once you're finished with your initial detox, it's important to continue to maintain a healthy digestion so that your body's ability to naturally eliminate toxins is not impaired. On a daily basis, you can start off your mornings with a glass of warm water with lemon and a bit of honey to improve elimination. Eat lots of fiber-rich foods like celery, split peas, and lentils. Supplement with probiotics, digestive enzymes like Papain, and liver-supporting herbs and supplements like Milk Thistle, ALA, NAC, and Glutathione (I'll get more in depth with these supplements in the following sections 2 & 6). Incorporate more detox-supporting foods in your diet like dark leafy greens, chlorella, wheatgrass, and seaweed. Do this, and you'll be well on your way to improving your digestion and your body's natural ability to eliminate toxins.

Step 2: Love Your Gut

Your gut is a complex environment in which both "good" and "bad" bacteria reside. Your gut plays a crucial role in your overall health, and has even been dubbed the body's "second brain," because of its tremendous impact on the brain and nervous system. Not only does your gut affect your brain, but it plays a critical role in maintaining healthy skin—and with over 100 trillion bacteria in the intestinal tract alone, it's no wonder why disruption in the gut would lead to other health issues. The gut is a delicate balance between the symbiotic relationship that occurs between the "good" and "bad" bacteria, and it can be thrown off with the consumption of poor foods, antibiotics, and even stress or lack of sleep. When the gut is functioning normally, it is able to properly digest food and extract the needed vitamins and minerals required for healthy skin. When the health in the gut goes awry and an overgrowth of the "bad" bacteria occurs, digestion is impaired and the skin suffers as a result. This microbial imbalance in the gut is referred to as "gut dysbiosis," and can lead to greater issues in the intestinal tract such as ulcerative colitis, irritable bowel syndrome, celiac disease, Crohn's disease, and SIBO (Small Intestinal Bacterial Overgrowth), all of which can contribute to poor skin. In fact, research has shown that nearly half of all acne suffers have an underlying gut imbalance that has not yet been resolved. If you frequently experience feeling bloated, fat, constipated, sluggish, mentally dull, fatigued, stressed, moody, suffer from headaches, have difficulty concentrating, or have digestive discomfort, there is a good chance you may have an imbalance in your gut. Try starting your mornings off with warm water and 2 tablespoons of lemon juice, followed by a fiber-rich breakfast or fiber supplement, and supplementing with a probiotic as well as digestive enzymes. If problems still persist, it might be in your best interest to visit a naturopathic doctor to figure out what the cause of your discomfort could be.

Improve Elimination

In addition to the tips I mentioned above, implementing the following tips can help improve your gut by improving the elimination of waste. A large majority of Americans are actually estimated to have anywhere from 3-11 pounds of waste stuck and left stagnant in their bodies! Talk about gross! It would appear that contrary to the popular children's book *Everybody Poops*, that not everybody is actually pooping. Not only is that an unpleasant thing to think about, but the health issues that can arise from such a problem can potentially be serious. Constipation is something that can cause you more than just a little abdominal discomfort, but can contribute to mental fog, bloating, toxicity, hemorrhoids, poor skin, and bacterial imbalances as well as their associated diseases like the ones previously mentioned. Here are some tips I would suggest for anyone seeking to improve their bowel movements, and ultimately improve their skin as a result!

1. Start your mornings off with a cup of warm water and 2 tablespoons of lemon juice. You can add 1 tablespoon of honey if you wish. Lemon is a natural detoxifying agent, and combined with the warm water it works to stimulate bowel function (especially when taken first thing in the morning).

2. Eat Fiber Rich Foods. Fiber helps move waste through the small and large intestines. One main reason people aren't effectively eliminating waste is because they consume a diet that lacks fiber. To get more fiber into your diet, simply eat more fiber-rich foods, or try supplementing with fiber pills or psyllium husk.

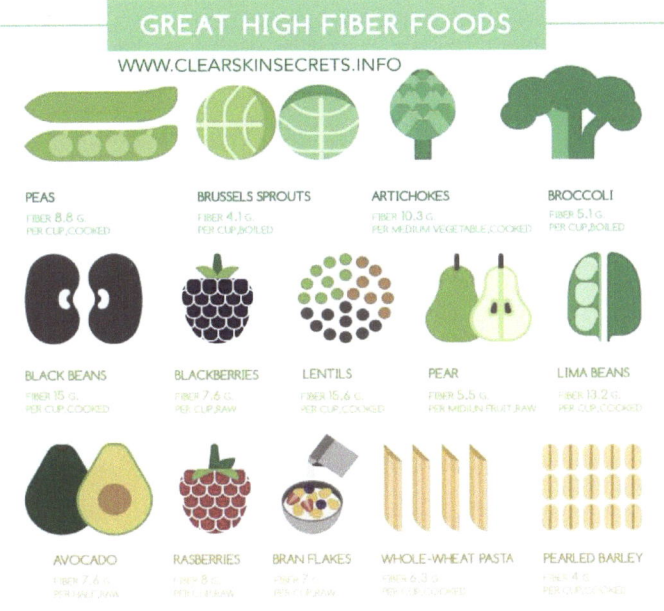

GREAT HIGH FIBER FOODS
WWW.CLEARSKINSECRETS.INFO

PEAS
FIBER 8.8 G.
PER CUP,COOKED

BRUSSELS SPROUTS
FIBER 4.1 G.
PER CUP,BOILED

ARTICHOKES
FIBER 10.3 G.
PER MEDIUM VEGETABLE,COOKED

BROCCOLI
FIBER 5.1 G.
PER CUP,BOILED

BLACK BEANS
FIBER 15 G.
PER CUP,COOKED

BLACKBERRIES
FIBER 7.6 G.
PER CUP,RAW

LENTILS
FIBER 15.6 G.
PER CUP,COOKED

PEAR
FIBER 5.5 G.
PER MEDIUM FRUIT,RAW

LIMA BEANS
FIBER 13.2 G.
PER CUP,COOKED

AVOCADO
FIBER 7.6 G.
PER WEDGE,RAW

RASBERRIES
FIBER 8 G.
PER CUP,RAW

BRAN FLAKES
FIBER 7 G.
PER CUP,RAW

WHOLE-WHEAT PASTA
FIBER 6.3 G.
PER CUP,COOKED

PEARLED BARLEY
FIBER 4 G.
PER CUP,COOKED

Fiber Rich Foods Include:

Celery, Wheat Bran, Oats, Peas, Brussel Sprouts, Artichokes, Raspberries, Avocados, Lentils, Beans, Brocolli, Blackberry, and, Barley.

Fiber-Filled Go-Green Smoothie

If you live a fast-paced life and are constantly on-the-go, or just want a quick way to get some fiber into your diet, I've got the smoothie just for you! I call it my Fiber-Filled Go-Green Smoothie! To make this smoothie you will need:

- 1 Rib of Celery
- 1 Pear
- 1 Green Apple (Juiced)
- 1 Avocado
- 1 Cup of Coconut Water

Simply blend the ingredients together and enjoy!

3. Supplement with probiotics and a digestive enzyme. Probiotics work to restore the "good" bacteria in the gut which help assist with the breakdown of food and digestive process. Digestive enzymes also aide in digestion and the breakdown of food. These are two supplements that can help improve symptoms of constipation, and can bring about an overall healthier gut.

4. Exercise. Many of us live in a very sedentary lifestyle which typically consists of sitting in a car to go to work or school, then sitting for hours on end at a desk, then sitting on the commute back home, and finally, sitting again in front of the television, computer, or book! The fact of the matter is that many of us just aren't getting the kind of movement our bodies need. If you want healthy, regular, and painless bowel movements, it's imperative that you get some physical movement into your day! Try at least 30 minutes of moderate exercise a day (or at least 3 times a week if your schedule is really too crammed).

5. Sleep More. Be sure to get enough sleep! Your body needs rest as a time to repair itself, restore itself, and also, to eliminate waste. If you aren't getting the rest you need (at least 8 hours of sleep), there's a good chance your body may struggle with digestive issues, including eliminating waste. Get enough sleep and you'll be doing your whole body a favor (and it will show in your skin!)

6. Drink Kombucha with Chia Seeds. I am a HUGE fan (and that's an understatement) of Kombucha and Chia seeds. The health benefits of the two are seemingly endless. Chia seeds are packed with more protein, more fiber than oatmeal, and more Omega 3's than salmon per serving. Kombucha has been found to be helpful in treatment of

tendonitis, arthritis, multiple sclerosis, kidney stones, asthma, allergies, bronchitis, it slows down aging, reduces wrinkles, improves memory, reduces fat, clears acne, increases libido, balances your pH, and naturally detoxifies. In addition to all of this, Kombucha is great for the skin because of its antioxidants as well as its antimicrobial probiotics. It also has a trace amount of caffeine as well as other minerals and nutrients that aide with the body's elimination of waste. The combination of fiber from the chia seeds and the Kombucha will get you going in no time!

I hope these tips help improve your digestion, and may you have some happy poops!

Eliminate Parasites

Part of "Loving Your Gut" includes getting rid of any "unwanted visitors." Many people are under the conception that contracting parasites can only occur through eating contaminated food, or traveling to a foreign country, however that is not the case. Parasites can be contracted through something as simple as touching a doorknob, walking around barefoot, or shaking hands with someone. It's been said before that approximately 90% of Americans suffer with a parasitic infestation and don't even know it. When our immune system is low, when we have high amounts of stress in our life, or a nutrient-deficient diet, we become even more susceptible to parasitic infestation.

Our colon is filled with good and bad bacteria, and when there is a lack of good bacteria, our body's ability to derive nutrients it needs from the foods we eat becomes impaired and our body suffers for it. One of the main problems caused by a parasitic infestation is Acne. Check out some of the other common symptoms below that having parasites (or an abundance of "bad" bacteria) can cause to see if parasites might be the root problem of the issues you're your skin:

-Skin Problems (Like acne)

-Gas/ Bloating (especially whenever you eat)

-Constipation

-Diarrhea

-Anemia

-Allergies

-Sleep Disturbances

-Chronic Fatigue

-Decrease Immunity

-Irritable bowel Syndrome

-Joint and Muscle Aches & Pains

If you've experienced some, any, or all of these symptoms, you might want to consult your doctor and request a blood or stool test for parasites. The good news is the problem is easy to fix. You can treat parasites by getting a low pressure colonic cleanse through a certified and experienced practitioner, taking probiotics, and supplementing with natural herbs and foods. Here is a list of herbs and super foods you can begin incorporating into your diet to help your body rid itself of any parasites:

-Pumpkin Seeds

-Garlic

-Pomegranate

-Quassia

-Southenwood

-Tansy

-Wormwood

-Neem

-Food Grade Diatomaceous Earth (Add 1 tsp to water and drink 30 minutes before eating)

These are all helpful foods and herbs to incorporate into your diet to get rid of parasites, but for a serious parasitic cleanse, I highly recommend **Dr. Clark Store's Cleansing Kit**, which consists of clove, green black walnut tincture, and a super-herb blend (and can be found on Amazon for $40). Once you complete the 2-week cleanse and get rid of the parasites, it's also important to do a follow-up treatment for the sake of maintenance. You can incorporate a Fresh Green Black Walnut and Wormwood Complex by "Now" (which can also be found on Amazon), as well as Yerba Prima's Psyllium husk, and Yerba Prima's Bentonite clay (also found on Amazon). Mix the clay and the husk into a drink and consume it once in the morning and once in the evening, followed by a glass of water. Wait 1 hour to take the "Now" parasite cleanse tincture, and then follow that with a glass of water. Wait another 15-30 minutes to eat. Also be sure to incorporate a probiotic to help your body produce more good bacteria so it can derive the nutrients it needs from the food that you eat. Probiotics are a necessary component of clear skin and they help us extract nutrients from our food and keep the "bad bacteria" in check. They are something I highly suggest to anyone seeking flawless skin.

For more information about parasites, check out the book "The Cure for All Diseases," by Hulda Clark.

Step 3: Balance Hormones

One reason that may be contributing to your break-outs is having a hormonal imbalance. Hormonal imbalances can result in symptoms like mood swings, food cravings, menstrual cramps, and, you guessed it... acne. But take heart! You need look no further for a solution to your unwanted problems. The answer to balancing hormones lies within the foods that we are eating. That's right, it's time to eat our ways to hormonal health so that we can supercharge our energy and libido, balance our hormones and mood, and consequently, feel good all month long and have clear and beautiful skin! If that sounds appealing to you, keep reading!

The information I'm about to share with you comes from Alisa Vitti's Woman Code: Perfect Your Cycle, Amplify Your Fertility, Supercharge your Sex Drive, and Become a POWER SOURCE!

While the information in this section is directed towards females (we have A LOT more going on hormonally) the information and dietary changes I'm about to share with you are helpful whether you are male or female. Men still go through hormonal fluctuations and changes too, even if they aren't as intense as the ones females experience.

If you still get your periods, you're going to want to start this change in your eating habits a day after your period is over. If you've already been through menopause, you can start dietary changes beginning the first Sunday of the month. If you're a man, you can begin these dietary changes also on the first Sunday of the month. Hormones affect everything we do, so regardless of whether or not you still get your period, it's important to make sure you're feeding your body according to what it needs.

Week 1: Sprouted & Fermented Foods

The first week after your cycle ends, you want to make sure you're providing your body with the nutrients it needs for increasing estrogen during this time. Sprouted and fermented foods are important because they're loaded with nutrients, prebiotics, and something known as "indole-3-carbinol" which helps the body break down and remove excess estrogen from the body. You'll want to eat things like: Kimchi, Sauerkraut, Broccoli, Sprouts, Bean, Alfalfa Sprouts, and Sprouted Ezekiel Bread.

Week 2: Raw Juices & Fresh Veggies

For your second week, it's necessary to have lots of raw vegetables and juices. You can make a juice with things like beets, kale, parsley, celery, lemon, and ginger. The possibilities are endless! The reason for this is because all of those vegetables are full of antioxidants and will help your liver produce more of the super-antioxidant, glutathione. Glutathione helps the break-down and removal of excess estrogen from our system. While it can be taken in supplement form, it's best to induce the natural production of it in our bodies by eating lots of fresh veggies. You can also boost your natural glutathione levels with supplements like N-acetyl-cysteine (NAC) and Alpha-lipoic-acid (ALA).

Week 3: Greens & Grains

During the third week after your period, estrogen and progesterone levels are fluctuating and are on the rise and fall. You'll want to eat lots of greens and grains like quinoa and buckwheat. These foods are low on the glycemic index and won't spike your blood sugar, and are also building blocks for seratonin, which will help keep your mood in check when Auntie Flo comes-a-knockin'.

It's also important to eat leafy greens like bock choy, escerol, and kale which have a high-fiber content to clean estrogen and remove waste from the body.

Week 4: Healthy Fats & Root Vegetables (full of vitamin A)

Lastly, during week four, you're going to want to eat healthy fats and root vegetables. Healthy fats help provide your body with what it needs to manufacture the hormones it needs while improving mood and restoring energy. Root vegetables (especially the orange ones): Pumpkin, yams carrots, and beets are all packed with Vitamin A. Vitamin A is needed in the liver in largely stored amounts so that estrogen can be broken down.

Step 4: Balance Blood Sugar

When I heard that another term for acne was "diabetes of the skin," my jaw dropped. Here I was wondering why I had such terrible skin, while stuffing my mouth with cookies, brownies, and other sweet vices. I had a blood-sugar imbalance. One of the key factors in helping me overcome my sugar addiction was Dr. Jacob Teitelbaum's highly informative book, *Beat Sugar Addiction Now!* (And I highly recommend it to anyone seeking more information on the subject). Our bodies crave sugar because it's a fast form of energy; however, it's not a healthy one.

It's been estimated that one third of the calories we consume come from sugar (and white flour which the body treats like sugar) that are added during food processing. About 140-150 pounds of sugar per person are added to our diets every year by food processors. In fact, sugar has been deemed "the cocaine of the food industry," and being the highly addictive substance that it is, giving you a temporary "high" but wreaking havoc on your body later, I couldn't think of a more appropriate name. The good news is, there are a few very simple things we can do to not only balance our blood-sugar levels and thus heal our skin, but to kick our sugar cravings to the curb for good!

#1: Drink Plenty of Water to Aid Sugar-Detoxing

Regularly drinking clean (non-tap) water, makes it much easier to kick your sugar cravings to the curb. Drinking water helps our bodies detoxify and rid ourselves of waste and things like unneeded, excess sugar. In addition, for those who crave sugar because of a hormone imbalance, drinking enough water helps aid hormone balancing. Make sure to frequently check if your lips or mouth are dry, or if your urine is a dark color. If you have any of those symptoms, it means you're dehydrated and need to start drinking more good quality (non-tap) water!

#2: Consistently Get a Good Night's Sleep to End Sugar Cravings

Poor Sleep -> Sugar Cravings -> Poor Skin

I want you to remember that poor sleep leads to sugar cravings, which leads to poor skin. If you don't get 7-9 hours of sleep a night, you will feel tired, and your body will begin to crave sugar as an attempt to create more energy. Because our bodies associate sugar as a source of instant energy, we crave it if we aren't getting replenished with energy when we sleep. If you want to beat your sugar cravings, make sure to get enough sleep so your body can get the restorative rest that it needs.

#3: Improve Your Nutrition: Switch from Junk-Food to Whole-Food

If you struggle with sugar addiction, and all the other issues that come along with it, like acne and fatigue, one of the best things you can do for yourself is to switch from a junk-food to whole-food diet. Eating whole foods means eating grains, nuts, fruits, and vegetables before they become processed (I'll discuss the best foods you can eat for your skin more in Step 7). When you eat junk food, your body will lack nutrients and as a result, you'll crave more sugar. Eating whole foods will help bring your body the nutrients it needs to optimally function, get rid of sugar cravings, and have clear skin once and for all!

#4: Supplement Intake to Defeat Sugar Cravings

One of the ways you can help overcome any sugar addictions is by adding supplements to your diet to naturally promote the production of energy and blood sugar balancing. Taking Chromium Picolinate and Cinnamon was one of the most beneficial things I did when it came to balancing my blood sugar. Not only did it help get rid of my sugar cravings and balance my blood-sugar, but I'm convinced it played a critical role in helping clear my skin. Here are a few more supplements to help balance your blood sugar and get rid of sugar cravings:

-Chromium— Chromium has been shown to balance blood sugar levels and even help diabetics. It can also help you lose weight and can cut out your desire or need for sugar because of the insulin balancing it brings. If you struggle with sugar addiction, this is a great supplement to incorporate in your daily diet.

-Licorice— Licorice can help slow down the breakdown of adrenal hormones, which means there will be more hormones available to help your body break down sugar. It can dramatically help reduce sugar cravings and even bring healing to the stomach.

-Vitamin D— Not having enough Vitamin D can increase the risk of suffering with depression, and can aggravate sugar cravings. By supplementing with vitamin D, you can raise the "happiness molecule," serotonin, which can alleviate depression and lessen the intensity of your sugar cravings. Taking a daily walk outside or reading out in the sunshine can help you get more Vitamin D, as well as supplementation.

- Vitamin B Complex— If you're the kind of sugar addict that lacks energy and turns to sugar for an energy boost, supplementing with B Vitamins is critical for energy production.

-Mulberries— This amazing super-fruit has been shown to lower glucose levels, reduce sugar spikes after consuming large amounts of sugar, reduce the risk of diabetes, and help get rid of sugar cravings. You can consume a mulberry supplement, tea, or eat fresh mulberries or dried mulberries in place of granola or have them as a crunchy snack. These are especially useful to have around if you know you're going to indulge in a little more sugar than usual.

-Nopal (Cactus) Supplement— Cactus has been found to be extremely helpful in the treatment of insulin and balancing blood sugar (as well as a number of other health benefits, like detoxing and lowering bad cholesterol). Supplementing with Nopal can improve your blood sugar and help beat sugar cravings. Health Force makes a great, vegan Nopal Supplement.

Just make sure to check with your doctor if you are diabetic or taking insulin.

#5: Exercise: Build Energy to Reduce Sugar Dependency

In our bodies, energy is created where energy is needed. When we exercise, our bodies need more energy, so more energy is produced, and as a result, we have more energy! When we exercise, we build more energy in our bodies, and we become less reliant on sugar to keep us going throughout the day. If you want to kick your sugar addiction, it's vitally important to exercise regularly. If exercise isn´ t your thing, start with 30 minutes of walking a day and work your way up. Your body will thank you for it!

#6: Cut Back on the Alcohol

There's nothing wrong with having a little alcohol in moderation, however if you notice it causes you to crave more sugar, you might consider cutting back on it. There is a cross addiction between sugar and alcohol, so if you find it causes you to crave more sugar, it's in your best interest to cut back.

Step 5: Boost Immunity

Our immune system is what prevents infection and fights off disease. It also plays a role in fighting off bacteria and maintaining healthy skin. When the immune system becomes compromised, it can result in a number of diseases and ailments, including acne. In order to prevent and treat acne, we must then address the immune system. I made this chart to outline what lowers immunity, versus what boosts the immune system. It's important to engage in as many immunity-boosting activities as possible, and to avoid activities that take a toll on our immune system if we wish to have clear and healthy skin.

Lowers Immunity	Boosts Immunity
Stress	Healthy Stress Management (Yoga, Meditation, Journaling, Counseling, Exercise)
Toxins	
Antibiotics	
Poor Diet	Detoxifying the Body
Lack of Sleep	Nutrient-rich, balanced Diet
Pollution	Getting enough Sleep
Depression, Emotional Issues	Supplementing (Zinc, Vitamin C)
Lack of Exercise	Positive thinking
	Engaging in Positive Experiences
	Drinking Plenty of Water
	Laughter

In addition, there are a few things you can begin to supplement with in order to boost your immunity, and they are: Vitamin C, Colloidal Silver (10 parts per million), Zinc (no more than 100mg a day), Echinacea, and Goldenseal (only take for a week at a time).

Step 6: Supplementation

In this day and age, much of our soil has become nutrient-depleted, so that even if we eat a completely healthy diet, we may still be missing some of the key nutrients that we need to maintain a healthy body and clear skin. This is where supplementation is incredibly helpful and important. All of the supplements I'm about to mention are essentials for healthy skin, and are so much safer than the prescription drugs used to treat skin problems nowadays.

Vitamin A with Beta- Carotene- Vitamin A strengthens the epithelial (skin) tissue. Beta-carotene is an antioxidant and precursor of Vitamin A.

Vitamin B- Is important for a healthy skin tone and works as an "anti-stress" vitamin. Extra Vitamin B3 improves blood flow to the surface of the skin. Deficiencies of Vitamin B3 have been linked to acne.

Vitamin C with Bioflavanoids- Promotes a healthy immunity and is needed for collagen and repairing of the skin tissue.

Vitamin D- Promotes healing and repair of the skin tissues.

Vitamin E- An anti-oxidant that enhances healing and tissue repair. (Use the D-alpha-tocopherol form).

Chlorophyll- Aids in cleansing the blood and preventing infections. It also supplies the body with key nutrients.

Kelp- Is rich in vitamins and minerals, especially B vitamins, which are essential for clear skin. It can help those with mineral deficiencies. Note: Kelp is also rich in iodine, which in some cases has been known to irritate acne symptoms. If you notice this, it may not be the supplement of choice for you.

Spirulina — An algae rich in vitamins and nutrients essential for skin-health. It's an antioxidant, anti-inflammatory, anti-bacterial, and antiviral.

*Garlic-*Destroys bacteria and works to enhance immunity.

Essential Fatty Acids (Primrose and Flaxseed oil)- EFA's supply the body with essential gamma-linolenic acid, which is needed to keep the skin smooth, soft, and supple, repair tissues, and dissolve fatty deposits that block pores. They also aid in healing the skin.

*Echinacea and Goldenseal-*Both are useful in the treatment of skin disorders and help boost the immunity. Note: Goldenseal cannot be taken for more than a week at a time and should not be taken by those who are pregnant, breastfeeding, have a history of cardiovascular disease, diabetes, glaucoma, or are allergic to ragweed.

Burdock Root and Dandelion Root —These are powerful blood and liver cleansers. When the liver is not functioning at its best, it has trouble breaking down excess hormones and as a result, can cause breakouts. These roots also contain inulin, which can improve the condition of the skin by removing harmful bacteria.

Milk Thistle —Blood and liver cleanser. Important for removing harmful toxins from the body that may cause imperfect skin.

Glutathione —Glutathione is a powerful antioxidant that is produced in the liver. It works to detoxify harmful compounds and excrete them out of the body. While some question the effectiveness of taking glutathione orally, it's production can also be induced by taking supplements like N-Acetyl Cysteine (NAC) and Alpha-Lipoic acid (ALA), both of which are powerful antioxidants and detoxifiers.

Selenium —A powerful anti-oxidant that also promotes skin elasticity.

L-cysteine —Contains sulfur which is needed for healthy skin.

Zinc —Aids in healing of the skin tissue, boosts immunity, and helps prevent scarring. Zinc is a necessary element in the glands that produce oil in the skin.

Probiotics —Replenish the essential bacteria needed to reduce acne outbreaks.

Additional Antioxidants which are great for the skin: *Green Tea, Grape Seed Extract, Pine Bark Extract (Pycnogenol) Bilberry Extract.*

My personal three favorite products that are incredibly healing and protective to the skin are The Beauty Chef's Glow Powder, Jane Iredale's Skin Acumax, and Isotonix OPC-3. All of which can be purchased online. Jane Iredale's Skin Acumax is like food for the skin, and I take double the dosage to ensure I get the correct amount of nutrients. Isotonix OPC-3 is a powerful, yet completely safe and effective blend of antioxidants. I take 3 times the dosage to really ensure I'm getting adequate antioxidant intake.

Moringa: The Super Seed

Moringa seeds are a truly amazing super seed that reap numerous health benefits for the body. In fact, the benefits are so extensive that I like to refer to them as "The Miracle Seed," as they've proven to be beneficial for digestion, bone health, brain health (improving the release of dopamine and serotonin), and have even been shown to aide in the treatment and prevention of diseases such as cancer and diabetes. Moringa seeds benefit the skin in a number of ways. They work to target several main issues involving the skin: Liver Health, digestive Health, and antioxidant levels. Moringa seeds protect the liver and boost the production of the antioxidant, glutathione. They are full of the antioxidants kaempferol, caffeoylquinic acid, zeatin, quercetin, rutin, chlorogenic acid, and beta-sitosterol, protecting the skin against toxicity, stress, and oxidative damage. They also improve digestion and protect the body against pathogens and harmful microbes. To reap the benefits of moringa for your skin, you need to simply take two seeds a day, followed by a glass of water. In addition, using Moringa oil on your skin can have wonderful healing benefits as well (which I'll share more about in the external care section).

Super Skin Healing Green Juice

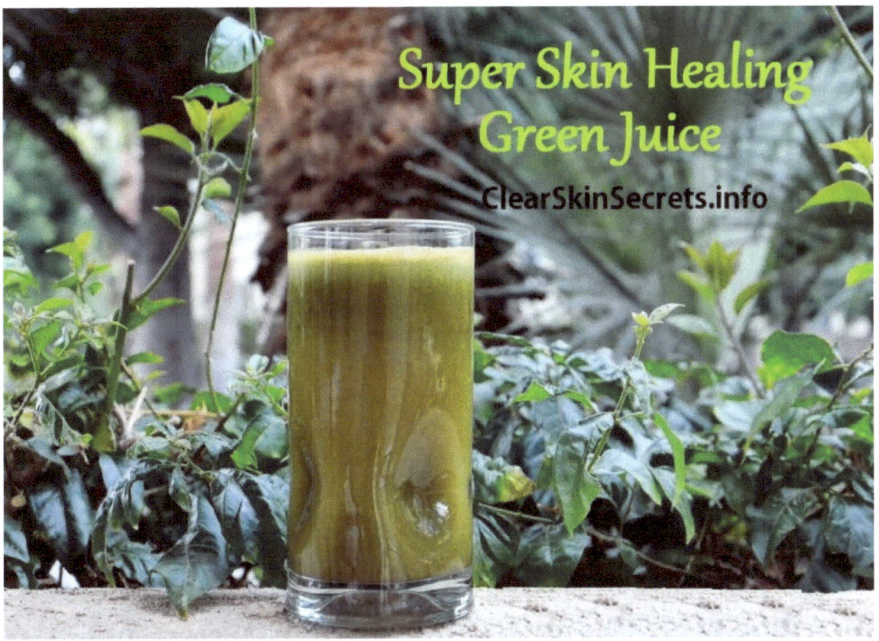

During the course of healing my skin, there was one main factor that was absolutely ESSENTIAL to my healing. It was drinking daily my own concoction of vegetables and herbs which I've come to call my "Super Skin Healing Green Juice!"

Now I'm warning you, this juice is quite tart and bitter, but it is so POWERFUL when it comes to healing the skin, that I think you'll agree, withstanding a little bitterness is quite worth it!

This Super Skin Healing Green Juice contains TWO highly potent, *highly healing* ingredients!

My two "secret" ingredients have been known to be extremely healing for the skin, curing ailments that range anywhere from acne, to psoriasis, to itching, to eczema. Additionally, they've been known to be powerful anti-oxidants, liver detoxifiers, and have even aided in the treatment of cancer and other chronic diseases. My recipe makes about 5 cups of juice, and because my two super-ingredients are potent and tart, this was the perfect amount of juice to water down their taste. If you'd like to make less juice, you can lessen the quantity of ingredients, (and if you'd like to make the juice less bitter, you can decrease the amount of healing herbs).

To make this *Super-Skin Healing Green Juice* you will need:

- 1 Cucumber
- 4 Carrots
- 1 stalk of Celery
- 1 handful of Parsley
- 1 handful of Cilantro
- 1 peeled Lemon
- 1 inch piece of Ginger

And my two *Super-Skin Healing Secret Ingredients* are:

- 1 tablespoon of Burdock Root Powder
- 1 tablespoon of Dandelion Root Powder

These two ingredients are powerful blood and liver cleansers. When the liver is not functioning at its best, it has trouble breaking down excess hormones and as a result, can cause breakouts. These roots also contain inulin, which can improve the condition of the skin by removing harmful bacteria.

If you suffer with any of the skin issues mentioned above (especially acne), I am almost CERTAIN that drinking this incredibly healing juice on a daily basis will clear them out!

The Beauty Smoothie

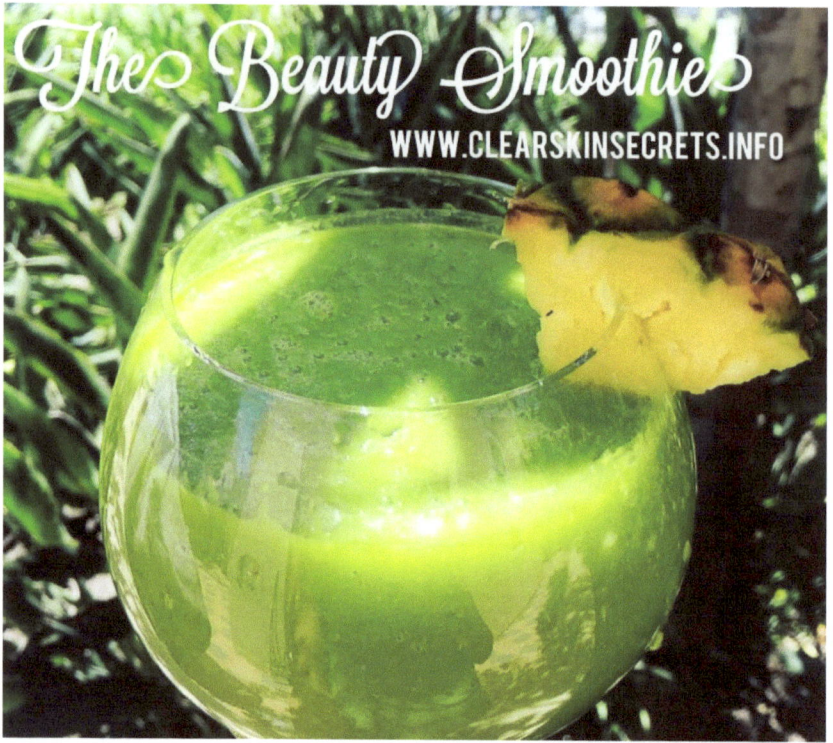

The following smoothie I'm about to share with you is full of key ingredients and vital nutrients necessary for maintaining healthy skin. I call it "The Beauty Smoothie," because it works to promote just that—beauty! For this smoothie, you will need the following ingredients:

- 1 Cup Spinach
- 1 Green Apple
- 1 Cucumber (peeled)
- 1 Avocado
- 1 Pineapple

Next you will need to juice the spinach, apple, and cucumber. Once you have the juice, blend it together with the avocado and the pineapple, and voila! You have yourself one delicious, healthy, and green Beauty Smoothie! The next step is to just sit back, relax, and enjoy!

Step 7: Diet and Lifestyle

There are several factors I have come to find are most important when maintaining a healthy lifestyle and having clear skin. In this section I'll discuss 4 Keys to a Healthy Lifestyle. This includes:

1.   The importance of having a whole-food, colorful, natural, and organic diet.

2.   Getting an adequate amount of sleep.

3.   Regularly exercising and having a healthy form of stress-management.

4.   Avoiding toxins in the household, environment, and social situations.

#1- Balanced Diet

Nutrients are essential to life, and they are especially essential to maintaining a healthy life. While supplementing with the vitamins and herbs I previously mentioned is important, consuming foods that are nutrient —rich and dense with things like fiber and minerals is equally important, if not even more-so important. It would do little good to be taking a variety of supplements, yet to still have a diet that is high-calorie, yet lacks nutrients. It would be counterproductive. Eating a colorful, wide-variety of fruits, nuts, vegetables, and grains is extremely important when it comes to having and maintaining clear skin. The reason for this is because the vitamins and nutrients we receive from our foods come in a much more *bioavailable* form for our bodies to digest. This simply means that the minerals and nutrients we receive from our foods come in a much more readily available and accessible form to be used by the body. The reason I also say it's important to eat a variety of colorful fruits and vegetables, is because each colored fruit and vegetable serves a different purpose. There are so many fruits, vegetables, and nuts that are packed with Vitamins A, E, C, and beta-carotene, all of which are essential to clear skin. Foods like Kale, Spinach, Dandelion Greens, Squash, Carrots, Sweet Potato, and dried Apricots are full of Vitamin A and Beta-Carotene. Vitamin E can be found in Spinach, Almonds, and Sunflower seeds. Oranges, Guavas, Kiwis, Yellow Bell Peppers, Strawberries, and Dark Leafy Greens like Kale are packed with Vitamin C which is vital to a healthy immunity. Dark greens like Chlorella, Spirulina, Wheatgrass, and sea vegetables like Kelp and Seaweed are necessary for removing harmful toxins from the body. Fruits and vegetables that are rich in anti-oxidants help prevent harmful toxins and free-radicals from causing damage to the body. Fruits and vegetables full of anti-oxidants include: Acai, Blueberries, Cherries, Cranberries, Blackberries, Strawberries, Prunes, Apples (Gala, Granny Smith, Red Delicious), Pecans, Plums, Walnuts, Hazelnuts, Kidney Beans, Pinto Beans, and Artichoke hearts. Each fruit and vegetable serves a different purpose, which is why it's so important to eat a wide variety of them. For your convenience, I've compiled a list of the fruits, vegetables, and nuts I just mentioned. While not every fruit and vegetable is on this list, it's important to know that anything you eat that came straight from the ground is good for you and important to eat if you desire clear skin. A good rule of thumb to go by, in the words of Michael Pollan: "If it came from a plant, eat it! If it was made in a plant, don't!"

Foods to Eat:	Foods to Avoid:
Greens: Kale, Spinach, Dandelion Greens, Chlorella, Spirulina, Wheatgrass, Kelp, Seaweed Berries: Blueberries,Strawberries, Blackberries, Cranberries, Acai, Cherries Fruits: Oranges, Guavas, Kiwis, Apples, Plums, Prunes, Dried Apricots Vegetables: Squash, Carrots, Sweet Potato, Russet Potato, Yellow Bell Peppers, Artichoke Hearts, Kidney Beans, Pinto Beans Nuts and Seeds: Almonds, Sunflower Seeds, Pecans, Hazelnut, Walnuts	Processed Sweets (Candy, Pastries, Cookies, Ice Cream) Junk Food (Pizza, Chips, Soda—Foods that are high in calories but low in nutritional value) Processed Foods (Anything that comes in a package) Fast Food Dairy Products (Butter, Cheese, Milk, Cream, Margarine) Eggs Alcohol Fried Foods

#2 Sleep

When it comes to maintaining clear skin, it's important to not only have a healthy diet, but a healthy lifestyle as well. Having a healthy lifestyle means getting plenty of sleep, so that your skin has time to restore itself. In fact, I cannot fully emphasize the importance of getting enough sleep, as sleep is the ONLY time the skin repairs itself. Sleep also helps keep the hormones and blood sugar levels balanced.

#3 Exercise & Stress Management

Exercise To Reduce Stress

Having a healthy lifestyle also means having a healthy form of stress management, such as journaling, and exercising, yoga, Zumba, or Pilates. Exercise is so important because not only does it help manage stress, but it also works to balance the blood sugar and eliminate toxins from the body. Which, as we've learned, are necessary components to maintaining clear and beautiful skin.

Meditate to Reduce Stress

Another great way to relax, "quiet," and ease the stress of the mind is to meditate. Meditation, though becoming increasingly popular, is something still very foreign and misunderstood by many people. When Buddha was asked, "What have you gained from meditation?" His apparent response was "Nothing! But let me tell you what I have lost: Anger, anxiety, depression, insecurity, fear of old age and death." That's a large claim, yet science is now just coming to new discoveries as to how beneficial meditation truly is for the body and mind. Meditation has been shown to work wonders by reducing stress and pain, relieving depression, increasing energy, productivity, memory, focus, and compassion, and restoring emotional balance. A few ways you can begin implementing meditation as a part of your life is to spend a few minutes (start at 5 and work your way up to 20) each day doing one of the following techniques:

-Focus on your breath- With each breath you take, count each inhale (1) and count each exhale (2) until you reach ten, then start over.

-Recite a mantra- Quietly recite a mantra, or a specific word or phrase that brings you a sense of peace and serenity.

-Guided Meditation- Guided meditation means directing your focus on visualizing an end goal. Many athletes do this to envision their victory before a race or game. Guided meditations can also be visualizations of you visiting a tropical beach, beautiful garden, or any other scenery which provides you with a sense of tranquility, peace, and joy.

-Focus on an Object- You can meditate with your eyes open, focusing on an object or icon that brings you peace or has significant meaning to you. If the object is not in front of you, simply close your eyes and visualize it in your mind. Not sure of what to visualize? Here are some ideas to focus on: The cross, the seed of life, the flower of life, a garden, the ocean, a flower, the stars, or a merkabah.

-Focus on your Body- This type of meditation requires that you be mindful of the different sensations you feel throughout your body. Notice any pain, tension, numbness, tingling, temperature, or relaxation you may be feeling, and focus on relaxing every muscle starting from the top of your head, down to your toes. This is a very mindful practice and will get you centered and in-the-moment.

Utilize Essential Oils to Reduce Stress

In addition to meditation and exercise, one of my favorite ways to relax and ease my mind is to put some essential oils in my essential oil diffuser and take a warm bath.

Essential oils have been known to have wonderful calming effects for many. They can be used to help achieve a calmer state of mind without the use of medications. You can add them to a massage lotion, dab a few drops diluted in water on your wrists, or put several drops in an essential oil vaporizer. Not only can oils have a calming effect, but they are said to help improve immunity and circulation as well.

Here are a few different essential oils as well as their healing effects on the mind:

Anti-Depressant ("Happy") Oils: **Basil, Clary Sage, Lavender, Lemon, Marjoram, Melissa, Peppermint, Vetiver, Ylang Ylang.**

Anti-Anxiety ("Calming") Oils: Basil, Melissa, Peppermint, Rosemary, Vetiver.

Mood Enhancing Oils: Bergamot, Chamomile, Clary Sage, Frankincense, Lemon, Melissa, Sweet Orange, Rose, Rosemary, and Sandalwood.

Please note that many essential oils cannot be used during pregnancy, and it's always wise to consult your health care practitioner before doing so.

#4 Avoid Toxins

Maintaining a healthy lifestyle also means you try to stay relatively clear of flooding your system with harmful toxins. This means avoiding processed foods, and things like tobacco, cigarettes, and alcohol. When you ingest these things, it puts a strain on your liver and digestion and is once again counterproductive to the efforts you make in eating healthy and taking supplements. I understand that drinking is a social thing, so if you go out with friends or to a party and feel you need something in your hand, try some grape juice, instead of wine, bottled kombucha instead of beer, or some tonic water with lemon instead of a gin and tonic. If you still feel the need to drink, remember moderation and maintaining balance is the key. So after a night of partying, simply use the next day to detox by exercising, and drinking some wheatgrass or beet, apple, and carrot juice. You'll feel good knowing that you're taking care of your body and preventing future problems by pushing it to its limits. It's also important to make sure you aren't unnecessarily inhaling or taking in toxins through the skin with the household cleaners or inorganic skin products. You can use baking soda and white vinegar as alternatives to harsh household chemicals. Natural alternatives to skin products I'll discuss more in Step 8.

Step 8: Balance Your Body's pH

What is pH and why should I care?

The pH or Potential of Hydrogen scale is what acidity and alkalinity are measured by. The foods and drinks we ingest alter the levels of our body's acidity or alkalinity. Things like certain drugs, as well as stress, sicknesses, and diseases can also throw off our pH balance.

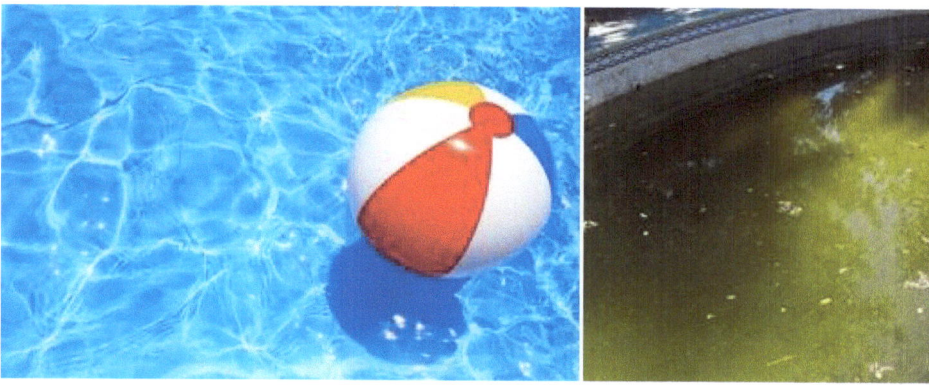

The pH of our bodies can be likened to that of a swimming pool's pH. Think of what happens when the pH of a swimming pool is out of balance: The water becomes green, murky, and gives off a funky smell. (Yuck!) If not treated quickly enough, moss can even begin to grow and the pool can become inhabited by mosquitos. When the pH of the pool is balanced however, the pool is clean, clear, and fresh crystal blue. (I don't know about you, but the balanced pH definitely sounds more appealing to me!)

In the same way, if pH imbalances go unaddressed in our bodies, it could lead to a variety of health issues: Including acne. The ideal pH for the body is between 7.35 and 7.45 (water is a neutral 7.0), making our internal bodies naturally slightly alkaline. However, normal skin pH is slightly more acidic, ranging from 4 to 6.5. This slightly acidic state creates the ideal environment in which skin cells can grow, function, and multiply. It also helps keep unwanted bacteria from clogging the pores and creating blemishes. When the skin's pH balance is off, we become more prone to break outs, and our skin's ability to repair and re-grow is impaired.

What Causes pH Imbalance?

Imbalances in our body's pH can be caused like things like poor diet, malnutrition, and stress. In addition to diet, imbalances in our skin's pH can be caused by things like using certain soaps or abrasive scrubs and exfoliates when cleansing the skin. The best way to keep the skin and body balanced is through diet, and by using non-abrasive skin products and natural cleansers like the ones I talk about in Step 9.

How to Keep the pH Balanced: The 80-20 Ratio

When it comes to maintaining a balanced pH, a rule of thumb you want to go by is maintaining a diet that consists 80% of alkaline-forming foods and drinks, and 20% acid-forming foods and drinks.

Here are a list of some of the acid-forming and alkaline-forming foods:

Acid-Forming Foods	Alkaline-Forming Foods
Alcohol	Avocados
Beans	Corn
Buckwheat	Dates
Chickpeas	Fresh Coconut
Cocoa	Fresh Fruit (most of them)
Coffee	Fresh vegetables (onions,
Cranberries	potatoes, rutabagas)
Legumes	Honey
Lentils	Maple syrup
Meat	Mushrooms
Milk	Onions
Oatmeal	Raisins
Olives	Sprouts
Pasta	Almonds
Prunes	Chestnuts
Sauerkraut	Lima beans
Soft Drinks	
Sugar	
Tea	
Vinegar	
Aspirin, Tobacco, and most drugs	

All vegetables, especially raw vegetables, help keep the body's acidity/ alkalinity in check. Even citrus fruits, though they seem acidic, help promote alkalinity. *One of the absolute best things you can do for your body and skin is to have a diet as full of as many raw fruits and vegetables as possible!*

Step 9: External Care

Now that I've addressed the internal aspect of treating acne, I'd like to address the external treatment of acne. There are certain things you want to avoid if you wish to have clear skin, like inorganic products that are animal tested, full of chemicals, preservatives, and other unwanted harmful substances that strip the skin of its natural and necessary oils. Our skin needs those oils to prevent dryness, premature aging, and damage. In order for acne to heal, you want the skin to be as clean as possible, as often as possible. This means avoiding the use of makeup whenever able to, and avoiding touching or picking at blemishes. This also means using organic, natural, non-comedogenic products that are as close to the earth as possible. Non-comedogenic means it is a product has been specially formulated as to not cause pore-blockages. When it comes to skin care, I don't even bother buying expensive creams or products. I simply cleanse my face with essential oils, natural astringents, makeup removers, and moisturizers, and fruit facial masks! All of these are completely harmless, and as close to nature as you can possibly get when it comes to skin care!

Seabuckthorn- Seabuckthorn is useful in the treatment of acne when taken internally or applied externally. Internally it helps boost the immunity, balance hormones, and reduce inflammation. When applied externally, seabuckthorn softens, soothes, and strengthens the skin, reducing inflammation, irritation, scarring, and swelling and is helpful in the treatment of acne as well as a variety of other skin disorders. Seabuckthorn comes in the form of oil which can be applied topically, and is also in many natural soaps that can be used for cleansing the skin. One of my favorite Seabuckthorn products is Living Libation's Best Skin EVER serum, which contains Seabuckthorn, Lavender, and other essential oils that are healing to the skin.

Lavender Oil- Lavender kills bacteria and stimulates new cell growth. It is a great antibiotic and antiseptic and can be directly applied to the individual blemishes.

Tea Tree Oil- A natural antibiotic and antiseptic. It can be used with just a few drops in water to wash your face with.
Vitamin E Oil- Vitamin E oil helps heal scars and retains skin moisture. You can buy the oil or buy them in capsule form and then break them open. Cleanse the face without drying it, and then apply the oil and leave on for 10 minutes before rinsing. For daytime use, use 5000 IU of Vitamin E for a less glistening effect.

Moringa Oil- Moringa oil is absolutely amazing! Not only does consuming moringa seeds have incredibly beneficial, healing properties for the skin, but applying the oil on your face has proven effective for treating acne as well! It has anti-aging properties, and works to effectively remove blackheads and pimples from the skin. It can be used as a natural cleanser, reducing redness, bacteria, and inflammation in the skin because of its antibacterial and anti-inflammatory properties.

Witch Hazel-When applied topically, witch hazel has astringent and healing properties. It also works to reduce itching and is a useful ingredient when it comes to skin care.

Rose Oil-A natural Antiseptic, Antibacterial, and Bactericidal, a few drops of rose oil can be added to water and used to cleanse the face.

Apple Cider Vinegar- Mix 1 part Apple Cider Vinegar with 10 parts water and apply to the affected area of skin. Doing this will help keep the skins pH balanced.

Sandalwood- An age-old Ayurvedic treatment for skin disorders, sandalwood works by removing excess oils and bacteria from the face that would normally cause breakouts. Sandalwood has antiviral, anticarcinogenic, and bactericidal properties. It can be purchased in oil form, or in a natural soap.

African Black Soap- African black soap is a natural cleanser and great alternative to the harsh chemicals found in stores. While it does not work to remove existing acne, it works by naturally removing the excessive oil and bacteria which caused the acne in the first place. All it consists of is cocoa pod, roasted plantain skins, palm kernel oil, coconut oil, palm oil and natural sodium. I use the soap made by Shea Moisture.

Raw Vegan Facial Masks

Not only do fruits and super-foods work amazing wonders on the skin when we consume them, but their vitamins, high-nutrient, and anti-oxidative qualities make them the perfect option for creating some wonderfully simple and amazing fruit facial masks! Certain fruits like papayas, pineapple, apples, grapes, and lemons are rich in Alpha-Hydroxy Acids (AHAs) which help to exfoliate the skin and remove dead skin cells that would otherwise clog the oil glands. Whether suffering with acne, dry skin, wrinkles or other pesky skin problems, (or if you simply want to maintain supple, healthy, and even-toned skin) using a quick and simple fruit mask can work wonders for your skin.

Why spend tons of money, or have to worry about harsh chemicals damaging your skin, when you can simply put fruit on your face to heal itself instead! My motto is, "If it's safe enough for you to eat, it's safe enough for you to put on your face!" I hope you enjoy this compilation of raw and edible, healing-skin fruit and super-food facials! Time to start a Himalayan salt or Lavender bath and treat yourself to a mini-spa day! Enjoy! :-)

Redness-Reducing Rose Water Cherry Mask

Use: Reduces blemishes and leaves skin looking smooth and radiant

Ingredients: Cherries and Rosewater

Application: Blend or mash several cherries, and add a few drops of rosewater. Spread thin layer on the face and leave on for 15 minutes. Rinse with lukewarm water and pat dry.

Acne-Scar Healing Apple Cider Vinegar Mask

Use: To reduce the appearance of acne scars. Apple Cider Vinegar and Tea tree oil act as a natural antiseptic and antibacterial. Calendula is incredibly healing for the skin.

Ingredients:

- 1/2 cup apple cider vinegar
- 1/2 cup raw organic honey
- 1/4 cup baking soda
- 1/4 cup of fine sea salt
- 10 drops of calendula oil (optional)
- 10 drops of tea tree oil (optional)

Application: Mix ingredients together and apply as a mask. Leave on your face for 3-4 minutes before rinsing off and patting dry.

Remarkably Radiant Red Apple Mask

Use: Leaves skin looking luminous and naturally glowing.

Ingredients: 1/2 Red Apple

Application: Blend apple and leave on skin for 15 minutes. Rinse with lukewarm water and pat dry.

Wonderful Watermelon Mask

Use: Nutrifying the skin, providing hydration, and acting as a natural exfoliant.

Ingredients: Watermelon pulp

Application: Spread a thin layer of the pulp on your face and neck. Leave on for 30 minutes or until dry, then rinse with cold water and pat dry.

Sinfully Smooth Skin Strawberry Mask

Use: Removes excess oil from the skin

Ingredients:

- 2 Strawberries
- 1-2 tsp honey

Application: Mash or blend the strawberries then apply on the face for 10-15 minutes. Rinse with lukewarm water and pat dry.

Orange You Beautiful Cleansing Mask

Use: Increase blood flow and provide nutrients to the skin.

Ingredients: Orange Pulp

Application: Spread pulp on face and neck. Leave on for 20 minutes then rinse off using cold water.

Perfect Skin Papaya-Mango Mask

Uses: Clears acne, Cleanser, Removes dead skin, Toner

Ingredients:

- Mango and Papaya Skin

Application: Flip the mango and papaya skin inside-out and massage onto your face. Let sit for 10-20 minutes. Rinse with warm water and pat dry.

Banana-Rama Resplendent Skin Mask

Use: Works as an emollient, softening and smoothing the skin
Ingredients:
- 1 ripe banana
- 1 tsp sandalwood
- 1-2 tsp honey

Application: Mix all of the ingredients then apply on the skin for 10-15 minutes. Rinse and pat dry.

Terrific Turmeric Anti-Inflammatory Mask

Uses: Anti-inflammatory, healing for the skin, reduces redness and visibility of acne.

Ingredients:

- 2 tsp chickpea powder
- 1 tsp olive oil

- 1/2 tsp turmeric
- 2 tsp water

Application: Mix all the ingredients and spread evenly over the face or affected area. Leave on for 10-15 minutes, then rinse and pat dry.

Healing Honey Matcha Mask

Uses: Clears acne, Reduces Wrinkles, Anti-Aging, and Anti-Inflamatory

Ingredients:

- 1 tablespoon of Honey
- 1/8 teaspoon of Matcha Green Tea Powder.

Application: Stir together and apply to face. Let sit for 10-20 minutes and wash off with lukewarm water.

Beautiful Skin Blue-Green Algae Mermaid Mask

Uses: Heals acne, Anti-Oxidant, Anti-Aging

Ingredients:

- 1 tablespoon of Aloe Vera Gel (from the plant, not processed)
- 1 tablespoon of RAW, organic honey
- 2 teaspoons of spirulina powder

Application: mix into a mask and allow to dry for 15-20 minutes, rinse with warm water and pat dry.

Honey Cinnamon Mask

Uses: Works as an Exfoliator or Moisturizer, Clears Acne

Ingredients:

- 1 Teaspoon of Honey
- 1 Teaspoon of Cinnamon

Application: Mix ingredients together until you get a thick paste. Apply and leave on for 20 minutes or overnight for severe or chronic acne. Be careful if you have sensitive skin, ask this mask is a little more of an abrasive exfoliant. Wash off with warm water and pat skin dry.

Antioxidant Rich Chocolate-Avocado Mask

Uses: Moisturizing, Antioxidant, Awakens dead Skin

Ingredients:

- 1/4 of Avocado and
- 1 teaspoon of Cacao (NOT cocoa)

Application: Combine ingredients and mix in a bowl. Apply to your face and let sit for 20 minutes. Rinse with warm water and pat dry.

Summary

I hope you've found all of the information I've shared with you to be helpful on your journey to clear skin. It is my greatest desire that you be fully healed, so that you can feel comfortable, radiant, and wonderful in your own skin. Here's a re-cap of what I've discussed, so that you can have a quick reminder, source of motivation, and periodic checklist, to assure that you are making all of the necessary steps in having clear skin. I wish you the best of luck on this journey, and I send all my love your way!

1. Start your mornings with some warm water and lemon to support daily elimination.
2. Take a probiotic and digestive enzyme to support healthy digestion and maintaining the digestive tract's "good" bacteria.
3. Supplement with herbs like Milk Thistle, Dandelion, and Burdock to support a healthy liver and detoxification.
4. Supplement with ALA, NAC, and Glutathione to support the liver and detoxification.
5. Avoid toxins like tobacco, cigarettes, alcohol, and other drugs, harmful household toxins, chemical-infused soaps and shampoos, and heavy metals.
6. Avoid eating processed sugars, junk food, fast food, and other unhealthy foods. Have a diet that is as colorful and natural as possible. Remember the words of Michael

Pollan, "if it came from a plant eat it, if it was made in a plant, don't!"

7. Have a nutrient-rich diet and supplement with Vitamins A, B, C, D, and E to support healthy, clear skin.

8. Drink plenty of water and be sure to get enough sleep. Doing this will help balance your hormones, beat sugar cravings, improve your immunity, help the body detoxify, and help the skin repair itself.

9. Exercise and have a healthy form of stress-management. This will keep harmful intestinal bacterial in check, will help boost your immunity, improve detox, and balance blood sugar.

10. Clean your face with products as close to nature as possible. Trade out inorganic products for ones that are closest to nature, like: Lavender Oil, Tea tree Oil, Seabuckthorn, and Witch Hazel.

For More Information

If you'd like to work with Brigitte one-on-one, or receive more helpful skin-healing tips, visit

www.ClearSkinSecrets.Info

www.ingramcontent.com/pod-product-compliance
Lightning Source LLC
Chambersburg PA
CBHW050811290526
45792CB00001B/72